Abnormal Labor

Causes and Management

Akmal El-Mazny

CONTENTS

	PAGE
− INTRODUCTION	1
− NORMAL LABOR	2
− MALPRESENTATIONS AND MALPOSITION	6
− OCCIPITO-POSTERIOR POSITION	8
− FACE PRESENTATION	10
− BROW PRESENTATION	12
− BREECH PRESENTATION	13
− TRANSVERSE PRESENTATION	16
− COMPOUND PRESENTATION	17
− CORD PRESENTATION AND PROLAPSE	18
− MULTIPLE PREGNANCY	20
− LABOR DYSTOCIA	24
− SHOULDER DYSTOCIA	28
− UTERINE RUPTURE	30
− CERVICAL LACERATIONS	33
− PERINEAL LACERATIONS	34
− POSTPARTUM HEMORRHAGE	36
− INTRAUTERINE GROWTH RESTRICTION	40
− PRETERM LABOR	43
− POSTTERM PREGNANCY	46
− PREMATURE RUPTURE OF MEMBRANES	47
− FETAL AND NEONATAL ASPHYXIA	49
− PUERPERAL PYREXIA	54
− THROMBOEMBOLISM IN PREGNANCY	58
− INDUCTION OF LABOR	61
− INSTRUMENTAL VAGINAL DELIVERY	63
− EPISIOTOMY	66
− CESAREAN SECTION	68
− REFERENCES	72

INTRODUCTION

The World Health Organization (WHO) defines normal birth as: spontaneous in onset, low-risk at the start of labor and remaining so throughout labor and delivery, the infant is born spontaneously in the vertex position between 37 and 42 completed weeks of pregnancy, and after birth, mother and infant are in good condition.

Abnormal labor constitutes any findings that fall outside the accepted definition of normal labor.

The three main factors associated with abnormal labor are the power (inadequate uterine contractions), the passage (abnormal pelvic anatomy), and the passenger (eg, macrosomia or malpresentation).

Abnormal labor suggests an increased risk of an unfavorable outcome, and alerts alternative methods for a successful delivery that minimize risks to both the mother and the infant.

This book provides a comprehensive review of abnormal labor along with its causes and management, which will be of immense value for obstetricians and allied health professionals.

NORMAL LABOR

Definitions

Labor is the physiological process by which a fetus is expelled from the uterus to the outside world.

Delivery means actual birth of the fetus.

The World Health Organization (WHO) defines normal birth as:

– Spontaneous in onset.

– Low-risk at the start of labor and remaining so throughout labor and delivery.

– The infant is born spontaneously in the vertex position between 37 and 42 completed weeks of pregnancy.

– After birth, mother and infant are in good condition.

Mechanism

Labor is achieved with changes in the biochemical connective tissue and with gradual effacement and dilatation of the uterine cervix as a result of uterine contractions of sufficient frequency, intensity, and duration.

The three main factors which affect the mechanics of active labor are

– The power (uterine contractions or maternal expulsive forces).

– The passage (pelvis or soft tissues).

– The passenger (the fetus).

Stages

The onset of labor is defined as regular, painful uterine contractions resulting in progressive cervical effacement and dilatation.

Labor is divided into three main stages that delineate milestones in a continuous process:

− The first stage (cervical dilation).

− The second stage (delivery of the fetus).

− The third stage (delivery of the placenta).

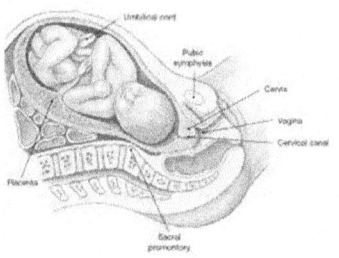

Pre-labor

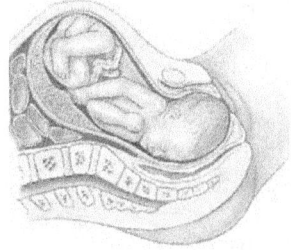

First Stage

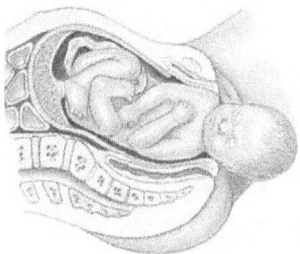

Second Stage

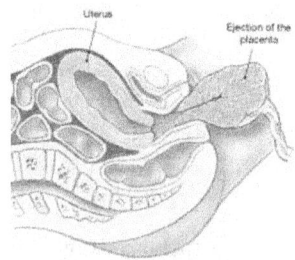

Third Stage

First Stage

—The first stage begins with regular uterine contractions and ends with complete cervical dilatation at 10 cm.

—The first stage is subdivided into an early latent phase and an ensuing active phase.

—The latent phase begins with mild, irregular uterine contractions that become progressively more rhythmic and stronger.

—This is followed by the active phase of labor, which usually begins at about 3-4 cm of cervical dilation and is characterized by rapid cervical dilation and descent of the presenting fetal part.

—The active phase is further divided into an acceleration phase, a phase of maximum slope, and a deceleration phase.

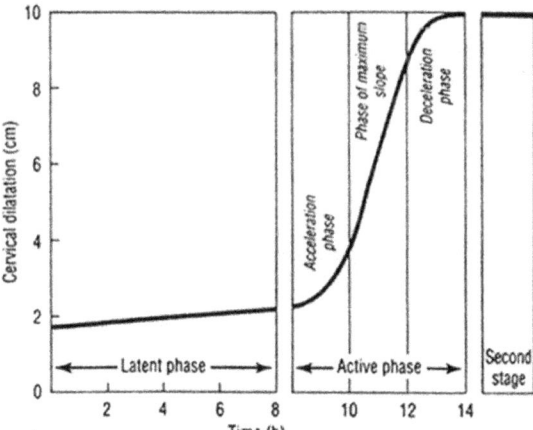

Second Stage

−The second stage begins with complete cervical dilatation and ends with the delivery of the fetus.

−For nulliparas, prolonged second stage of labor should be considered when the second stage exceeds 3 hours with regional anesthesia or 2 hours in the absence of regional anesthesia.

−In multiparous women, such a diagnosis can be made if the second stage of labor exceeds 2 hours with regional anesthesia or 1 hour without it.

Third Stage

−The third stage of labor is defined by the time period between the delivery of the fetus and the delivery of the placenta and membranes.

−The third stage of labor is considered prolonged after 30 minutes, and active intervention, such as manual extraction of the placenta, is commonly considered.

MALPRESENTATIONS AND MALPOSITION

Definitions

Lie

The relationship of the long axis of the fetus to that of the mother.

It may be longitudinal, transverse or oblique.

Presentation

The portion of the fetus that is foremost or presenting in the birth canal.

Malpresentations

All presentations of the fetus other than the vertex:

−Face.

−Brow.

−Breech.

−Transverse.

−Compound.

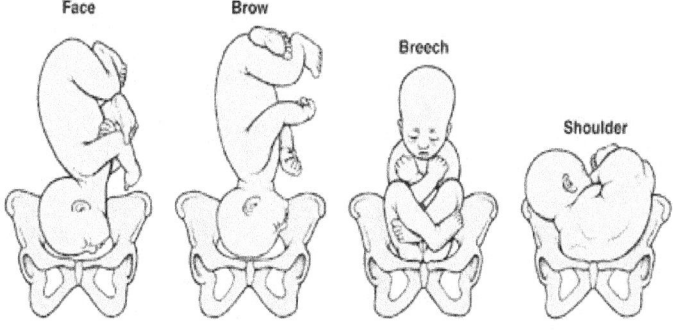

Position

Reference point on the presenting part, and how it relates to the maternal pelvis.

Normal position is occipito-anterior position (OA): when the fetal occiput is directed towards the mother's symphyisis or anteriorly.

Malposition

Occipito-posterior (OP): when the fetal occiput is directed towards the mother's sacrum or posteriorly.

Causes

−Defects of the power: laxity of the abdominal muscles, exaggerated dextrorotation of the uterus.

−Defects of passage: contracted pelvis, android pelvis, pelvic tumor, uterine anomaly, placenta previa.

−Defect of passenger: preterm fetus, macrosomia, multiple pregnancy, polyhydramnios, anacephaly and hydrocephaly, IUFD.

OCCIPITO-POSTERIOR POSITION (OP)

It is a vertex presentation in which the fetal back is directed posteriorly.

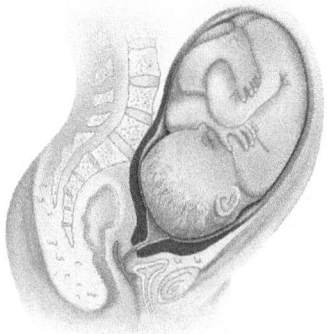

Diagnosis

Vaginal Examination

– The anterior fontanelle is palpated.

– Identify the sagittal suture which is mostly asymmetric.

– Dilation is often asymmetric, you can feel the fetal ear and a persistent anterior cervical lip is common.

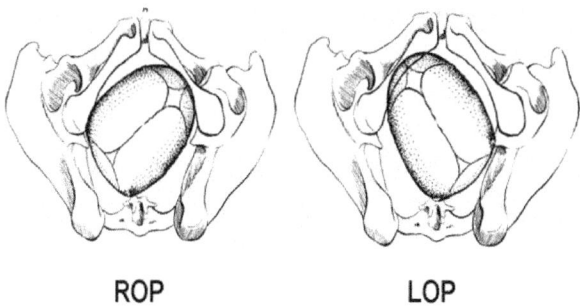

ROP   LOP

Management

– Spontaneous delivery is possible: make sure uterine contractions are adequate and no fetal distress.

– Manual rotation.

– Vacuum extraction delivery.

– CS should always be the backup method of delivery for any occipito-posterior presentation that cannot be safely delivered vaginally.

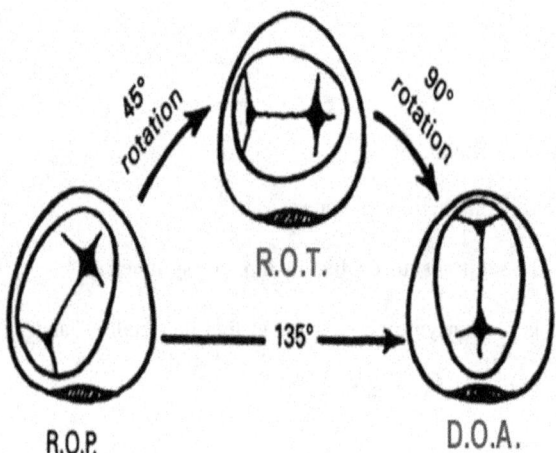

FACE PRESENTATION

Cephalic presentation in which the head is fully extended.

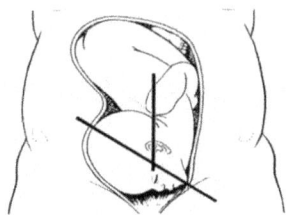

Diagnosis

Vaginal Examination

– The face is palpable and the point of reference is the chin; you should feel the mouth and be careful not to confuse it with breech presentation.

– It is necessary to distinguish the mento-anterior position from mento-posterior position.

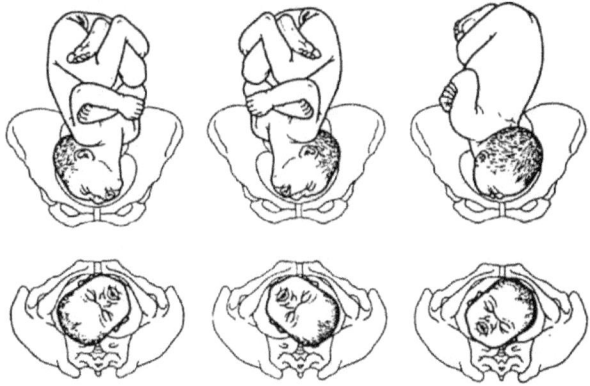

Management

Mento-anterior Position

−If the cervix is fully dilated: vaginal delivery.

−If there is slow progress and no sign of obstruction: augment labor.

−If descent is unsatisfactory: perform a CS.

Mento-posterior Position

−Deliver by CS.

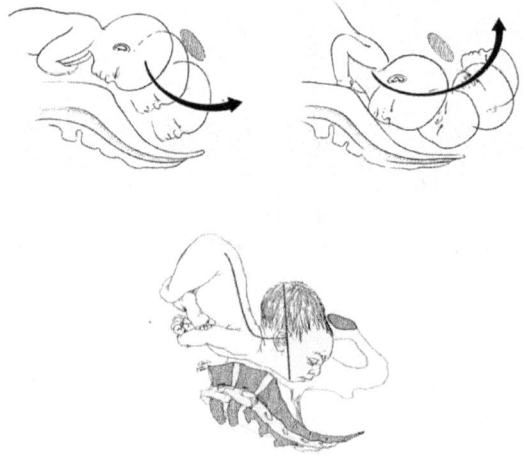

Face Presentation, direct mento-posterior
vaginal delivery is impossible.

BROW PRESENTATION

Cephalic presentation in which the head is midway between flexion and extension.

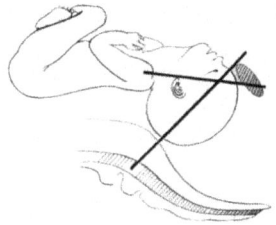

Diagnosis

Vaginal Examination

– The anterior fontannel and the orbital notches are felt; the referral point is the nasal apex.

– The chin is not felt.

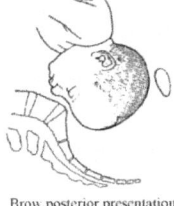
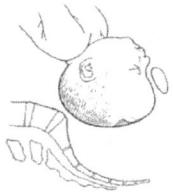

Brow posterior presentation   Brow anterior presentation

Management

– Deliver by CS.

BREECH PRESENTATION

Longitudinal lie in which the buttocks and/or the feet are the presenting part.

Types

−Complete (flexed) breech: both legs are flexed at the hips and the knees.

−Frank (extended) breech: both legs are flexed at the hips and extended at the knees.

−Footling breech: a leg is extended at the hip and the knee.

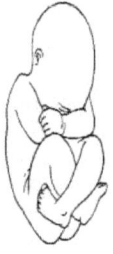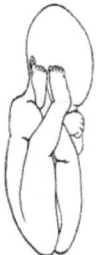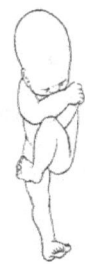

Diagnosis

Abdominal Examination

−The head is felt in the upper abdomen.

−The breech in the pelvic brim.

Vaginal Examination

−The buttocks and/or feet are felt.

−Thick dark meconium is normal.

Complications

−Entrapment of the after coming head.

−Nuchal arm.

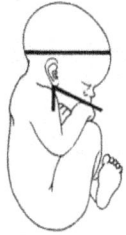 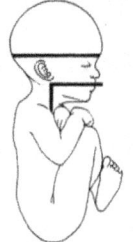 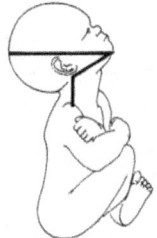

Management

External Cephalic Version

Consider at 37 weeks if all requirements are met:

−Adequate amniotic fluid.

−Placenta in fundal position.

−No uterine anomalies.

−No previous uterine scar.

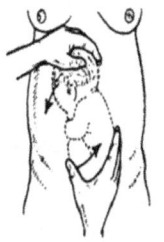 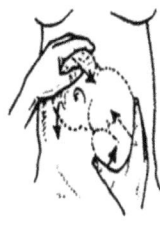 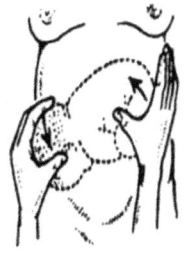 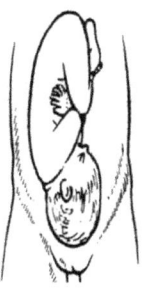

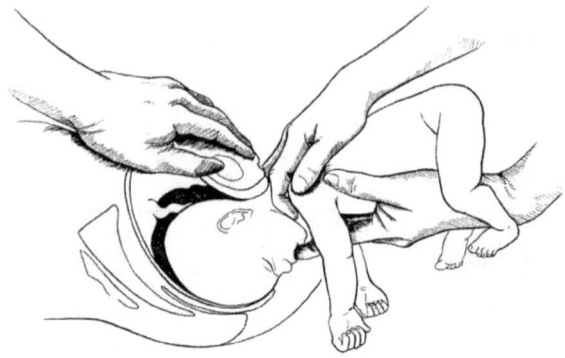

<u>Indications for CS</u>

− Primigravida.

− Footling breech.

− Hyperextension of fetal head.

− Nuchal arm.

− Macrosomia.

− Severe prematurity, IUGR, placental insufficiency.

− Other indications for CS.

TRANSVERSE PRESENTATION

Longitudinal axis of the fetus does not coinside with that of the mother.

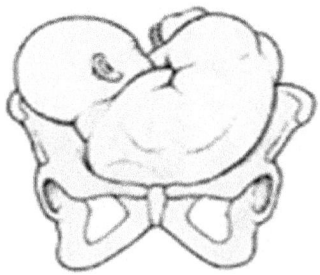

Diagnosis

During Pregnancy

− Inspection: abdomen is broader from side to side.

− Palpation: the fundus feels empty and the fundal level is lower than

  expected.

− Ultrasound confirms the diagnosis.

During Labor

− On vaginal examination, the scapula is felt as point of reference.

− Ultrasound confirms the diagnosis.

Management

− Deliver by CS.

COMPOUND PRESENTATION

Occurs when an arm presents alongside with the presenting part.

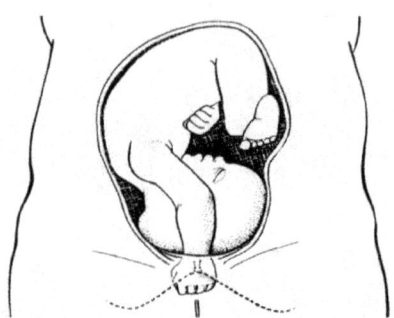

Diagnosis

Vaginal Examnation

−Fingers/arm is felt with the presenting part.

Management

−Replace the arm and if sucessful continue with viginal delivery.

−If cord prolapse: deliver by CS.

CORD PRESENTATION AND PROLAPSE

Definitions

−Cord Presentation: umbilical cord lies below the presenting part with intact membranes.

−Cord Prolapse: umbilical cord lies below the presenting part with ruptured membranes.

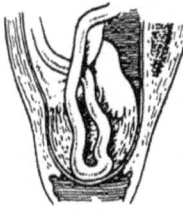 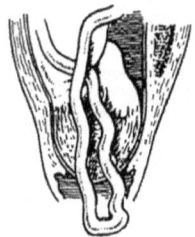

Cord Presentation   **Cord Prolapse**
Membranes Intact   **Membranes Ruptured**

Causes

−Long cord.

−Breech, shoulder, and other malpresentations.

−Contracted pelvis.

−Preterm labor +/- low birth weight <2500 g.

−Polyhydramnios.

−Multiple pregnancy (usually the second twin).

−Placenta praevia.

Diagnosis

−Feeling of a soft usually pulsatile structure on vaginal examination.

−Fetal distress.

Management

Pulsating Cord

−Delivery by CS is the safest method.

−Rarely, with a fully dilated cervix, deliver the head immediately by the forceps or the vacuum extractor.

Non-pulsating Cord

−If the foetus is certainly dead, labor is left to continue until eventual vaginal delivery.

MULTIPLE PREGNANCY

Definition

More than one fetus in the uterus.

Mostly twin pregnancy but others may be encountered, triplets or plus.

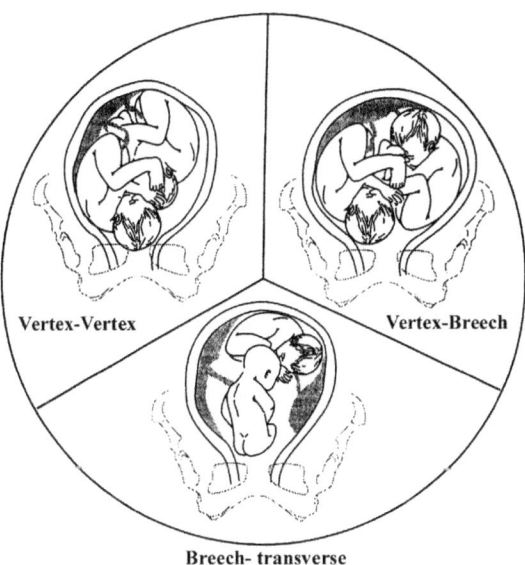

Vertex-Vertex   Vertex-Breech

Breech- transverse

Causes

− Ovulation induction.

− Assisted reproductive techniques.

− Hereditary factors.

− Previous multiple pregnancy.

Diagnosis

−Exaggerated symptoms of pregnancy.

−Fundal height larger the gestational age.

−Two audible fetal heart beats.

−Multiple fetal parts or more than two fetal poles.

Investigations

−Ultrasound to determine chorionicity.

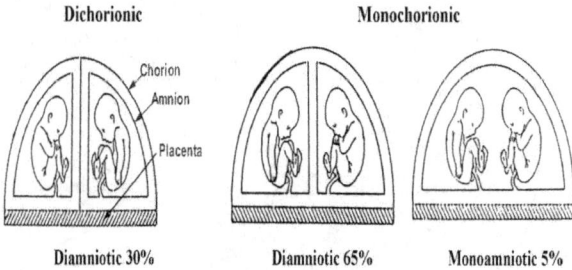

Dichorionic   Monochorionic

Chorion
Amnion
Placenta

Diamniotic 30%   Diamniotic 65%   Monoamniotic 5%

Complications

−Increased risk of miscarriage.

−Prematurity.

−Intrauterine fetal growth retardation.

−Fetal transfusion syndrome (twin-twin transfusion syndrome).

−Malpresentations.

−Pregnancy induced diabetes.

−Pregnancy induced hypertension.

– Antepartum hemorrhage.

– Postpartum hemorrhage.

– Polyhydramnios.

– Premature rupture of membranes.

Management

Antenatal

– Bed rest.

– Increase nutrition.

– Routine antenatal care.

– Ultrasound to determine presentation of first twin, detect anomalies.

– Monitor for associated obstetric complications.

Vaginal Delivery

– The first twin is cephalic.

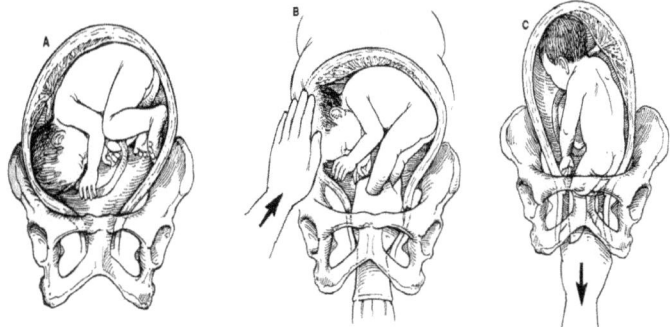

Delivery of the second twin (transverse lie) by Internal podalic version (IPV)
and vaginal breech extraction

<u>Cesarean Section</u>

− The first twin is not cephalic (locked twin).

− Retained living second twin.

− More than two fetuses.

− Previous uterine scar.

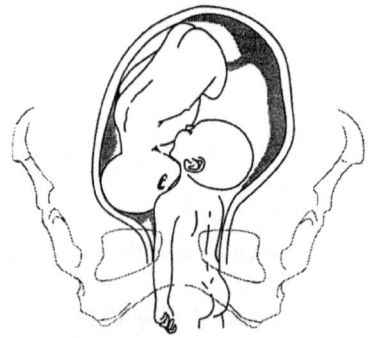

Locked Twin

<u>Third stage</u>

− Look for and anticipate postpartum hemorrhage.

LABOR DYSTOCIA

Definition

Dystocia of labor is defined as difficult labor or abnormally slow progress of labor.

Causes

–Power (inadequate uterine contractions, contraction ring of the uterus, myomas, uterine scar)

–Passage (abnormal pelvic anatomy)

–Passenger (macrosomia, malpresentation, malposition, fetal anomalies)

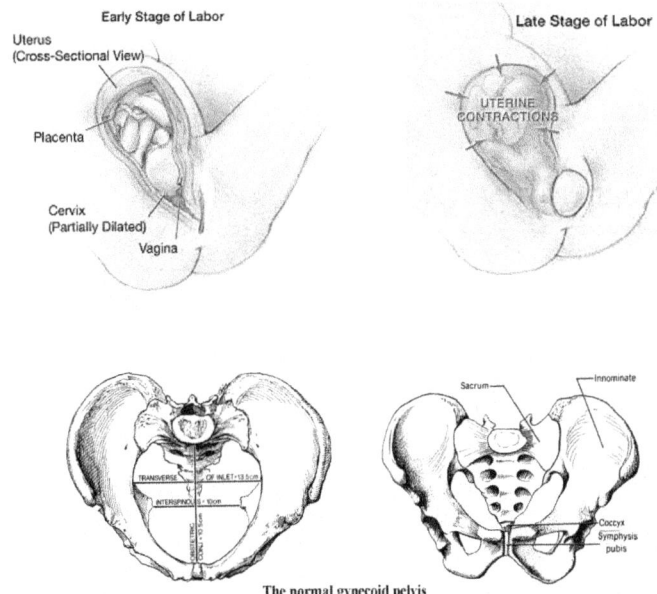

The normal gynecoid pelvis

Diagnosis

−Lumbar and abnormal back pain due to ineffective contractions.

−Dehydration.

−Anxiety.

−Failure of cervix to dilate despite good uterine contractions.

−Edema of the cervix and vulva.

−Failure of the fetal head to descend.

−Bandl's ring

−Fetal distress.

−Arrested labor.

−Maternal exhaustion.

Investigations

−Fetal monitoring with a partogram.

−Ultrasonography.

Complications

−Fetal distress.

−Fetal hypoxia / asphyxia.

−Fetal death.

−Rupture of the uterus.

−Birth canal injuries (cervical tears, vaginal and perineal lacerations).

−PPH.

−Postpartum endometritis.

−Maternal death.

Management

−Evaluation of uterine power, pelvis, passenger, pain.

−Fetal monitoring.

−Active management:

Pattern	Primi	Multi	Management
Prolonged latent phase	>20h	>14h	Stripping, Amniotomy, Prostaglandins or oxytocin (according to Bishop score)
Active phase, arrest of dilation	≤1.2cm/h	≤1.5cm/h	Stripping, Amniotomy or oxytocin, If no success – CS
No cervical dilation	≥2h	≥2h	Stripping, Amniotomy or oxytocin, If no success – CS
Arrest of descent in second stage	≥1h	≥1h	Stripping, Amniotomy or oxytocin, If no success – CS

−Correction of malposition: occipito-posterior position is significant contributor to dystocia; can be corrected by spontaneous rotation, manual rotation or by vacuum / forceps.

−Failure should prompt a CS.

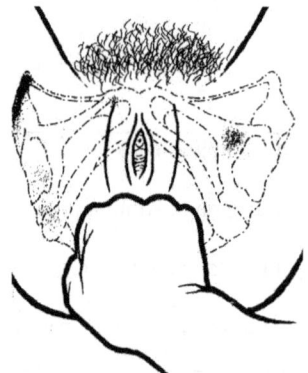

External Pelvimetry

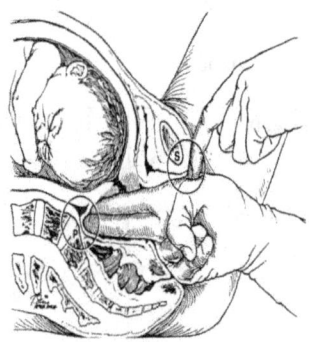

Internal Pelvimetry

SHOULDER DYSTOCIA

Definition

The fetal shoulders fail to deliver shortly after the fetal head.

Causes

−Fetal macrosomia.

−Diabetes.

−Maternal obesity.

−Age >35.

−Short in stature.

−Abnormal pelvis.

−Postterm pregnancy.

Diagnosis

−A prolonged first or second stage of labor.

−Turtle sign: appearance and retraction of the fetal head.

−Head bobbing in the second stage.

−Failure to restitute.

−No shoulder rotation or descent.

Complications

−Fetal injury (such as brachial plexus injury) and fetal death.

−Maternal injuries and postpartum hemorrhage.

Management

− Ask for help of an obstetrician, for anesthesia, and for pediatrics for subsequent resuscitation of the infant.

− Episiotomy.

− McRoberts' maneuver: hyperflexing the mother's legs tightly to her abdomen +/- suprapubic pressure.

− Rubin maneuver or posterior pressure on the anterior shoulder, which would bring the fetus in an oblique position with head somewhat towards the vagina.

− Woods' screw maneuver which leads to turning the anterior shoulder to the posterior and vice versa.

− Manual delivery of posterior arm.

UTERINE RUPTURE

Definition

Uterine rupture refers to a tear or separation of the uterine wall.

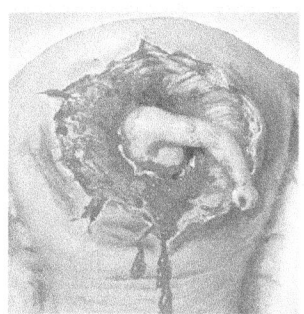

Causes

− Multiparity.

− Previous uterine scar.

− Malpresentation and malposition.

− Misuse of uterotonics.

− Placenta insertion anomalies.

− Contracted pelvis.

− Obstructed labor.

− Uterine manoeuvers.

− Instrumental deliveries.

− Trial of labor after CS.

Diagnosis

−Pre-rupture bandle ring sign.

−Sudden, severe abdominal pain (may decrease after rupture).

−Bleeding − intra-abdominal and/or vaginal.

−Cessation of uterine contractions.

−Tender abdomen.

−Absent fetal heart activity.

−Easily palpable fetal parts on the abdomen.

−Rapid maternal pulse.

−Hypovolaemic shock most of the time.

Investigations

−Full blood Count and blood group crossmatch.

−Clotting profile.

−CTG monitoring.

−Ultrasound in a stable patient (In cases of uterine dehiscence suspicion).

Complications

−Fetal demise.

−Uterine multi-laceration leading to Hysterectomy.

−Bladder laceration.

−Maternal death.

Management

Management of Shock

−Senior obstetrician, pediatrician and anaesthetist for assistance.

−Assess for clinical signs of shock e.g. cool, clammy, pale, rapid pulse, decreased blood pressure.

−Insert 2 large intravenous accesses using 14-16 gauge cannulas with appropriate intravenous fluid.

−Order 2-4 units of packed red cells.

−Administer oxygen via face mask 6L/min.

−Ensure the woman remains with her legs bent or in lithotomy to perfuse the brain.

Emergency Laparotomy

−Conservative or hysterectomy and repair complications (bladder or ureter tear…).

−If conservative, contraception for at least 2 years.

−Elective CS for the next pregnancy at 39 weeks of gestation or if uterine contractions start.

CERVICAL LACERATIONS

Causes

−Improper use of oxytocin and /or prostaglandins.

−Faulty application of forceps or ventouse.

−After coming head in breech presentation.

−Obstructed labor.

−Some cases of precipitate labor.

−Previous cervical cerclage.

−Placenta previa.

Complications

−PPH.

−Extension of the tear upwards into the lower segment or broad ligament.

−Infections.

−Incompetent cervix.

Management

−Management of shock.

−Suturing should start above the apex of cervical tear.

PERINEAL LACERATIONS

Definition

Tears of the perineal tissue between the vagina and rectum.

Grades

− 1st degree injury to perineal skin.

− 2nd degree injury involving perineal muscles but not the anal sphincter.

− 3rd degree involvement is of the anal sphincter.

− 4th degree involvement of the anal sphincter and anal mucosa.

Causes

− Assisted delivery.

− Prolonged secong stage of labor.

− Nulliparity.

  Macrosomia.

− Occipito-posterior position.

Complications

− PPH.

− Injury to bladder, uterus.

− Anal incontinence.

− Infections.

− Dyspareunia.

Management

−Surgical repair of the tear.

−Repair of the external anal sphincter end to end and internal inner sphincter should be repaired by interupted sutures.

−Repair of the 3rd and 4th perineal tear should be done in theatre under general or regional anesthesia.

−Its recommended to repair perineal tears with vicryl 2-0 which causes less irritation and discomfort.

−Check the anal canal if it is not closed during the repair.

−Antibiotics and laxatives are recommended to be used after anal sphincter repair.

−Women with history of anal sphincter injury in previous pregnancy who are symptomatic should be advised about elective CS.

POSTPARTUM HEMORRHAGE (PPH)

Definition

−Loss of more than 500 ml of blood from the genital tract in the first 24 hours after vaginal delivery and more than 1000 ml after CS.

−Excessive vaginal bleeding resulting in signs of hyovolemia (hypotension, tachycardia, oliguria, light headedness).

−A 10% decline in postpartum hemoglobin concentration from the antepartum levels.

Types

−Primary: within first 24 hours.

−Secondary: after 24 hours to the end of puerperium.

Risk Factors

−Overdistension of the uterus (polyhydramnios, multiple pregnancies, macrosomia…).

−Grand multiparity.

−Previous history of PPH.

−Antepartum hemorrhage.

−Myomatous uterus.

−Hypertensive disorders.

−Drug use (MgSo4, salbutamol…).

Causes

−Atonic uterus (70%)

−Genital tract trauma (20%)

−Retained placenta or placental fragment (10%)

−Coagulopathy (1%)

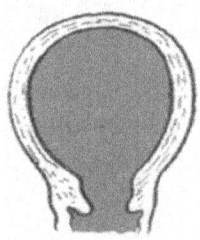

Atonic Uterus

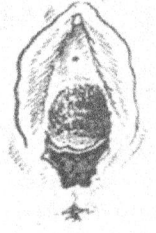

Genital Tract Trauma

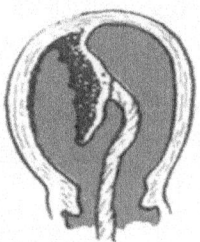

Retained Placenta

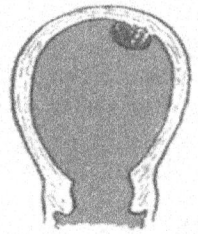

Retained Placental Fragment

Diagnosis

−Continuous vaginal bleeding.

−Signs of hypovolemic shock.

−Signs of anemia.

Complications

−Hypovolemic shock.

−Sheehan syndrome.

−Renal failure.

−Anemia.

−Death.

Management

−Call for help (obstetrician, anesthesist…).

−Resuscitation of the mother.

−Identification of the specific cause of PPH.

−Atonic uterus: bimanual compression and ecbolics (oxytocin, methyl ergometrin, misoprostol).

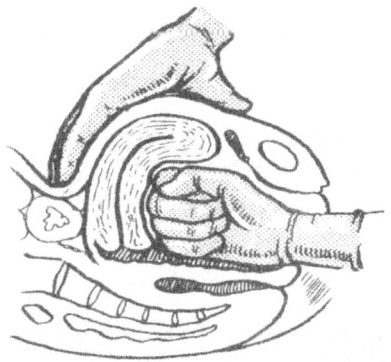

Bimanual Compression of the Uterus

- Genital tract trauma: vaginal exploration and repair under anaesthesia.

- Retained placenta or placental fragment: manual removal under anaesthesia.

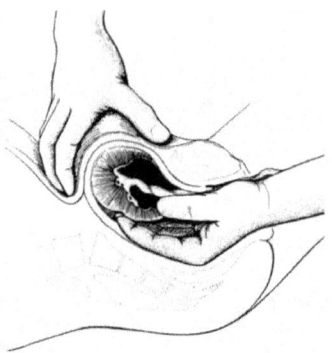

Manual Separation of the Placenta

- Coagulopathy: fresh frozen plasma, fresh blood transfusion, cryoprecipitate, fibrinogen, and platelet concentrate.

- If bleeding persists: internal iliac artery ligation or hysterectomy (standard procedure if bleeding is uncontrollable).

INTRAUTERINE GROWTH RESTRICTION (IUGR)

Definition

Intrauterine growth restriction (IUGR) or small for gestational age (SGA) is a fetal weight that is below the 10th percentile for gestational age as determined by ultrasound.

Types

– Symetrical.

– Asymetrical.

Causes

Maternal Factors

– Preeclampsia.

– Diabetes in pregnancy.

– Anaemia.

– Chronic hypertension.

– Poor nutrition.

– Cardiac disorders.

– Coagulopathies (thrombophilias).

– Respiratory disease (severe asthma…).

– Renal disease

– Anti-phospholipid syndrome.

Fetal Factors

−Fetal infection.

−Multiple pregnancy.

−Malformations.

−Chromosomal defects.

Placental Factors

−Decreased uteroplacental blood flow.

−Placenta praevia.

−Thrombosis, infarction (fibrin deposition).

−Placental cysts, chorioangioma.

Uterine Factors

−Fibromyoma (large submucosal fibroids).

−Uterine abnormalities - especially uterine septum.

Diagnosis

−Small fundal height for gestational age.

−Symptoms of the cause (diabetes, Preeclampsia...).

−Ultrasound findings <10th percentile estimated fetal weight.

−CTG.

−Biophysical profile.

−Umbilical artery Doppler.

Complications

−Fetal distress / IUFD.

−Meconium stained liquor.

Management

−Proper pregnancy dating.

−Treatment of the etiology.

−If end diastolic flow is present: delay delivery after 37 weeks.

−If end diastolic flow is absent, baby >34 weeks: consider delivery.

−Baby <34 weeks, patient should be admitted and monitored by CTG, receiving corticosteroids and consider delivery after 48 hrs by CS.

−If vaginal delivery, continous CTG is a mandatory.

−Suctioning pharynx as soon as possible after delivery to avoid meconium aspiration.

PRETERM LABOR

Definition

Preterm labor is occurance of uterine contractions before 37 weeks of gestation.

Causes

−History of previous preterm birth.

−Adolescent age and advanced maternal age.

−Maternal infections (pyelonephritis, genital tract infection, other systemic infections...).

−Increased uterine size (twins, poly hydramnios).

−Maternal trauma.

−Uterine abnormalities (myomas, malformations).

−Other pregnancy complications (abruption placentae, cervical incompetence...).

−Social, economic and stress factors.

Diagnosis

−Pelvic and back pain.

−Uterine contractions.

−Increased vaginal discharge / leaking of amniotic fluid.

−Muco-bloody discharge.

Investigations

− Vaginal swab for analysis.

− Urine analysis.

− Materanl and fetal screening for infections.

− Obstetric ultrasound.

Complications

− Prematurity.

− Neonatal respiratory distress syndrome.

− Neonatal mortality and morbidity.

Management

Cervix Dilatation <4 cm

− Tocolysis with calcium channel blockers (Nifedipine) or B2 agonists (Ritodrine HCL and Terbutaline sulfate).

− Monitor maternal heart rate (it should not go up 120/ min).

− Dexamethasone 6mg IM 4 doses 12 hourly for lung maturity.

− Delivery should be delayed for 24 to 48 hours.

Cervix Dilatation ≥ 4 cm

− Tocolyse with B2 agonists or Nifedipine for 24 hours.

− Dexamethasone 12mg IM 2 doses 12 hourly.

− This will assist transfer to a center with good neonatology facilities.

<u>During Labor</u>

−Continuous electronic monitoring of preterm fetus during labor is mandatory because preterm infants tolerate hypoxia more poorly than term infants.

−Avoid prolongation of the 2nd stage of labor.

−Episiotomy: to minimize head compression and decrease intracranial haemorrhage.

−CS is indicated in preterm breech, and the extremely LBW fetus.

−Neonates should be transferred to neonatology unit.

−Next pregnancy is at high risk for preterm labor and should be monitored closely.

POSTTERM PREGNANCY

Definition

Pregnancy lasting beyond 42 weeks from the first day of the LMP.

Causes

− Error in dating.

− Primiparity.

− Anencephaly.

Investigations

− Ultrasound.

− Umbilical artery Doppler.

Complications

− Fetal distress / meconium stained liquor.

− Dysmaturity syndrome.

− Fetal macrosomia.

Management

− Proper pregnancy dating.

− Induction of labor if no contraindication.

− CS if failure of induction or fetal distress.

PREMATURE RUPTURE OF MEMBRANES (PROM)

Definitions

−Premature Rupture of Membranes (PROM): rupture of fetal membranes 1 hour or more prior to onset of labor.

−Preterm Premature Rupture of Membranes (PPROM): rupture of fetal membranes 1 hour or more prior to onset of labor prior to 37 weeks.

Causes

−Maternal infections (pyelonephritis, genital tract infection).

−Cervical incompetence.

−Increased uterine size (twins, polyhydramnios).

Diagnosis

−Sudden gush of fluid from the vagina followed by intermittent trickle.

−Sterile speculum examination to confirm leaking of amniotic fluid.

−Nitrazine test to detect the alkaline pH of amniotic fluid in the vagina.

Investigations

−Full blood count.

−Vaginal swab for analysis.

−Urine analysis.

−Materanl and fetal screening for infections.

−Obstetric ultrasound.

Complications

−Infection (chorioamnionitis, neonatal sepsis, maternal septicemia).

−Prematurity.

−Neonatal respiratory distress syndrome.

−Neonatal mortality and morbidity.

Management

Termination of Pregnancy (irrespective of gestational age)

−Clinical and laboratory evidence of chorioamnionitis.

−Fetal condition is not reassuring.

PROM (>37 weeks)

−Termination of pregnancy under cover of suitable antibiotics and close
  fetal monitoring.

−Spontaneous labor will start within 24-48 hours in 80-90% of cases.

PPROM (<37 weeks)

−Prophylactic antibiotics given to guard against infection.

−Corticosteroids in cases <34 weeks.

FETAL AND NEONATAL ASPHYXIA

Definition

Fetal asphyxia is a state of inadequate oxygenation and inadequate elimination of CO2, which may result in metabolic acidemia (umbilical arterial blood pH <7.2).

Causes

Maternal Factors

−Maternal Age >40 years or <16 years.

−Pregnancy induced hypertension or preeclampsia.

−Diabetes.

−Severe anemia.

−Renal disease.

−Infections.

−Use of narcotics.

Fetal Factors

−Multiple pregnancy.

−Prematurity.

−Post term.

−IUGR.

−Macrosomia.

−Congenital malformation.

−Oligohydramnios and polyhydramnios.

−Hydrops fetalis, intrauterine infections and isoimmunisation.

−Non-reassuring fetal heart rate.

Pregnancy and Labor Factors

−Fetal distress.

−Antepartum hemorrhage.

−Postterm pregnancy.

−Prolonged PROM.

−Malposition and malpresentation.

−Meconium-stained liquor.

−General anesthesia.

−Instrumental delivery.

−Emergency CS.

Diagnosis

−CTG (tachycardia, bradycardia, late deceleration, variable deceleration).

−Mucous, blood or meconium in airway.

−No breathing seen or felt.

−No pulse felt at umbilical cord or no heart beat heard with sthetoscope.

−APGAR <7 at the 1st minute of life.

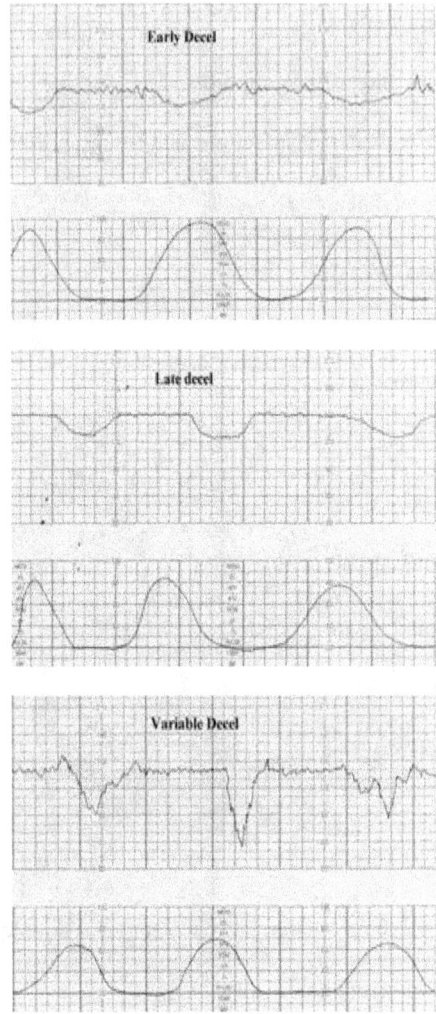

Complications

−Cerebral palsy.

−Neonatal death.

Management

Proper Antenatal Care

– Treat the probable cause of intrauterine asphyxia if possible.

Proper Intranatal Care

– Careful observation of CTG.

– Avoid operative trauma.

– Episiotomy especially for breech and premature infants.

– Aspiration of mucus and meconium from fetal larynx before breathing.

Clearing Air Passages

– Holding the infant from the feet.

– Aspirating mucus from mouth and upper pharynx by a rubber catheter.

Warming the Infant

– To decrease oxygen requirements.

– To avoid attacks of apnea.

Oxygen Therapy

– Small mask or stream in front of the mouth and nose.

– Endotracheal tube if indicated.

Artificial Respiration

– Endotracheal tube with intermittent positive pressure insufflation.

– Mouth to mouth breathing until endotracheal tube is available.

Cardiopulmonary Resuscitation:

- Cardiac resuscitation together with endotracheal entubation (or mouth to mouth breathing) if no audible heart beats or heart rate <100.

- Thumbs are put at the junction of lower and middle 1/3 of sternum to compress the chest gently 100 times per minute.

Pharmaceutical Management

- Adrenaline 0.01-0.03 mg/kg IV, IM, ET.

- Naloxone 0.1 mg/kg IV, IM, SC, ET if narcotic analgesia was used during labor.

- Normal Saline 10 cc/kg IV over 5-10 minutes.

- Dextrose 10% 2 ml/kg.

- Treat the underlying cause after stabilization, and refer the infant to neonatology unit.

PUERPERAL PYREXIA

Definition

Oral temperature of ≥38°C in the first 10 days postpartum or ≥38.7°C during the first 24 hrs postpartum.

Causes

−Benign fever.

−Endometritis.

−Breast engorgement.

−Mastitis/Breast abscess.

−UTI.

−Pneumonia.

−Wound infection (CS, cervical, vaginal and perineal lacerartions, episiotomy, uterine rupture).

−Deep venous thrombophlebitis.

−Pulmonary embolism (PE).

−Septic pelvic vein thrombosis.

−Pelvic peritonitis.

−Pelvic abscess.

−Malaria.

−Other causes of fever.

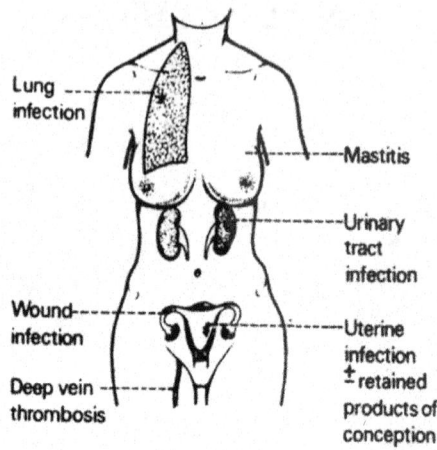

Risk Factors

−Increased duration of active phase of labor.

−Multiple pelvic examinations.

−Labor for ≥6 hours after ruptured membrane.

−Chorioamnionitis.

−Retained placenta or membranes.

−Urethral catheterization.

−Previous UTI.

−Operative vaginal delivery.

−Long operative duration.

−Anemia.

Diagnosis

−Fever.

−Sweating, tachypnoea, tachycardia.

−Chills.

−Headache.

−Malaise.

−Pelvic pain.

−Foul-smeeling lochia.

Investigations

−CBC, CRP..

−Urinary analysis with culture and sensitivity

−Wound swab for culture and sensitivity.

−Blood cultures.

−Cervical and uterine sample and sensitivity.

−Ultrasound.

−Doppler ultrasound for DVT.

Complications

−Puerperal sepsis.

−Peritonitis.

−Septicemia.

Management

− Complete aseptic measures.

− Avoid early rupture of membranes.

− Avoid multiple vaginal examinations.

− Isolation of suspected cases.

− Light nutritive diet.

− Frequent measurements of vital signs.

− Antibiotics: a combination of antibiotics (cephalosporins, gentamycin, and metronidazole) is given till the results of culture and sensitivity are obtained.

− Analgesics.

− Antipyretics.

− Treatment of complications.

THROMBOEMBOLISM IN PREGNANCY

Definitions

− Deep Vein Thrombosis (DVT) is the formation of blood clots within the deep veins, most commonly in the lower extremities or pelvis.

− Pulmonary Embolus (PE) is thrombosis or showers of emboli in the pulmonary vessels.

Pregnancy-associated Causes

− Changes in local clotting factors.

− Mechanical impedance of venous return.

− Vessel damage during pregnancy.

Risk Factors

− Advanced maternal age.

− Increased parity.

− Multiple pregnancy.

− Surgery (CS, episiotomy, lacerations...).

− Prolonged immobility.

− Dehydration.

− Prior DVT or PE.

− Lupus anticoagulant.

− Preeclampsia.

Diagnosis

−Pain or tenderness, fever.

−Asymmetric limb swelling, >2 cm larger than opposite side.

−Warmth or erythema of skin over area of thrombosis.

−Homans sign (calf pain with dorsiflexion of the foot).

−With PE tachycardia, dyspnea and chest pain.

−Death with massive PE.

Investigations

−Full blood count.

−Coagulation test (PTT, PT/ INR).

−Liver function, renal function.

−Ultrasound, Doppler.

−CT scan.

−Chest X-ray.

−Angiography.

Complications

−Septic pelvic thrombophlebitis.

−Death.

−Recurrent PE.

−Pulmonary hypertention.

Management

−Bed rest.

−Graduated elastic compression stocking should be applied.

−Inferior vena cava filter can be used to avoid PE.

−Enoxaparin: 1 mg/kg SC every 12 hours for the acute phase.

−Warfarin 5-7.5 mg loading dose and then the maintainence dose will depend on INR results for 6 weeks.

−Acetylsalicylic acid (aspirin): 75-100 mg daily to be continued up to 6 weeks postpartum.

−Enoxaparin can be substituted with heparin.

−Avoid hormonal contraception; risk increases with oestrogen containing contraceptions.

−For the next pregnancy, anticoagulation therapy throught pregnancy.

INDUCTION OF LABOR

Definition

- Stimulation of uterine contractions prior to the onset of spontaneous labor for vaginal delivery after the age of viability.

- The condition of the cervix (Bishop score) is the most important factor in successful induction.

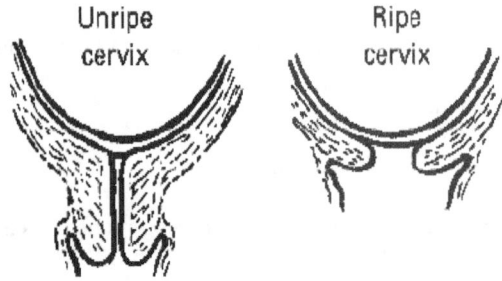

Unripe cervix   Ripe cervix

Indications

- Maternal medical conditions (diabetes, hypertensive disorders...).

- Postterm pregnancy.

- Intrauterine growth restriction.

- Intrauterine fetal death.

- Premature rupture of membranes.

- Chorioamnionitis if no contra indication.

- Isoimmunization.

- Fetal malformations.

Management

Misoprostol (PGE2)

− 50 mcg PO or intravaginal every 3-6 hours up to 6 times.

− Continously Monitor fetal heart rate by CTG after administration.

− Vaginal examination before the next dose.

Oxytocin (Bishop's Score >6)

− Oxytocin 5 IU in Ringers lactate or Normal Saline 500 ml

− Start with **8** drops/min then add 4 drops every 30 minutes, maximum 40

   drops/min

Artificial Rupture of Membranes (ARM) + Oxytocin

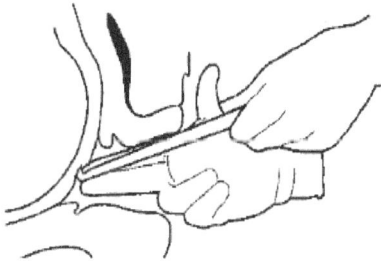

INSTRUMENTAL VAGINAL DELIVERY

Definition

Operative vaginal delivery is extraction of baby with use of instruments (obstetric forceps and vacuum extractor).

Indications

Fetal

−Fetal distress.

Maternal

−Prolonged second stage of labor.

−Maternal exhaustion.

Prerequisite for Instrumental Delivery

−Full dilatation of cervix.

−Engagement of fetal head.

−Empty the urinary bladder of the patient.

−Favorable presentation (vertex, deflexed vertex or face presentations).

−Vacuum extraction is contraindicated for face presentation.

−Vaccum extraction is contraindicated before 34 weeks of gestation.

−Instrumental delivery with high suspicion of failure should be done in theatre ready for CS.

−Episiotomy is not routenly indicated with instrumental delivery.

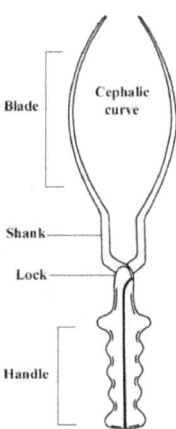

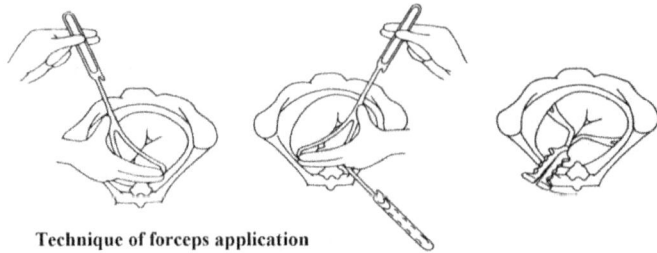

Technique of forceps application

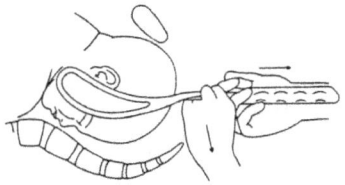

Direction of traction

Obstetric Forceps

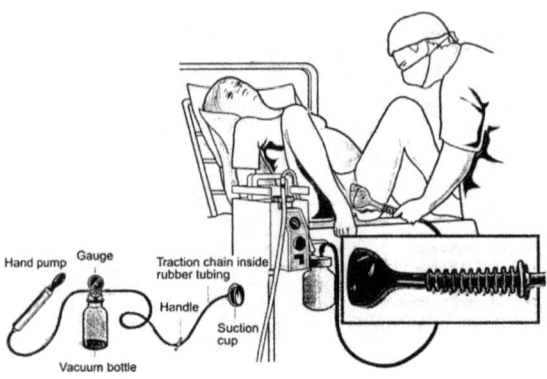

Vacuum Extractor

Complications

Maternal

− Traumatic injury including anal sphincter and bladder damage.

− Postpartum hemorrhage.

Fetal

− Skull fracture and/or intracranial hemorrhage.

− Cephalhematoma.

− Facial nerve injury.

− Facial skin bruises and lacerations.

EPISIOTOMY

Definition

It is an incision in the perineal body at the time of delivery.

Types

−Mediolateral episiotomy.

−Median episiotomy.

Mediolateral

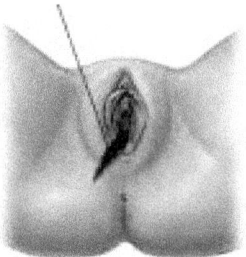

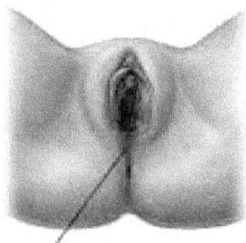

Median

Indications

−To prevent a tear (episiotomy is easier to repair).

−Previous perineal or pelvic floor repair.

−Contracted pelvic outlet.

−Face to pubis delivery.

−Vaginal breech delivery.

−Shoulder dystocia.

−Oversized foetus.

Complications

−Bleeding.

−Extension into anal musculature or rectal mucosa causing fecal incontinence.

−Fistula formation.

−Hematoma.

−Infection with suture disunion.

−Dyspareunia.

Management

−Repair as in perineal tear (2nd Degree).

−Post-episiotomy hygiene education.

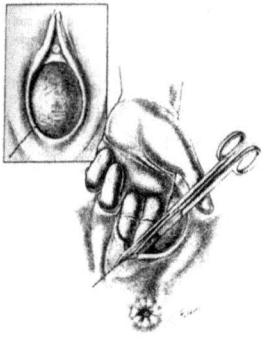 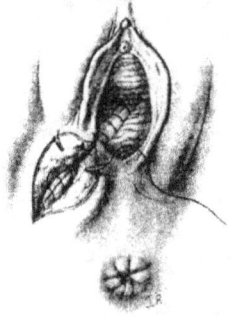

CESAREAN SECTION (CS)

Definition

Delivery of the fetus, placenta and membranes through abdominal and uterine incisions.

Indications

Maternal

−More than 1 previous cesarean delivery.

−Contracted pelvis.

−Obstructive tumors.

−Active genital herpes virus.

−Elective CS.

−Abdominal cerclage.

−Reconstructive vaginal surgery, eg, fistula repair.

−Medical conditions, eg, hypertensive disorders, diabetes mellitus, cardiac, pulmonary, thrombocytopenia.

Fetal

−Non-reassuring fetal heart pattern.

−Malpresentations.

−Cord prolapse.

−Macrosomia, congenital anomalies, multiple pregnancy.

Maternal-Fetal

−Obstructed labor.

−Placenta praevia (complete).

−Placental abruption.

−Perimortem.

−Maternal-fetal disproportion.

Complications

−Hemorrhage and shock.

−Urinary tract injury.

−Gastrointestinal injury.

−Anesthesic complications.

−Lacerations.

−Post operative peritonitis.

−Endometritis.

−Paralytic ileus, acute gastric dilatation, and intestinal obstruction.

−DVT and PE.

−Abdominal adhesions.

−Intrauterine synechia.

−Uterine dehiscence in the next pregnancy.

−Risk of uterine rupture for the next pregnancy.

Management

Pre-operative Management

− Anesthesia consultation: regional anesthesia is preferred than general anesthesia.

− Monitoring vital signs.

− NPO when elective CS.

− Intravenous: ringer lactate or normal saline 500 ml.

− Antibiotics.

− Urinary bladder catheterization.

− Laboratory investigations.

− Patient consent.

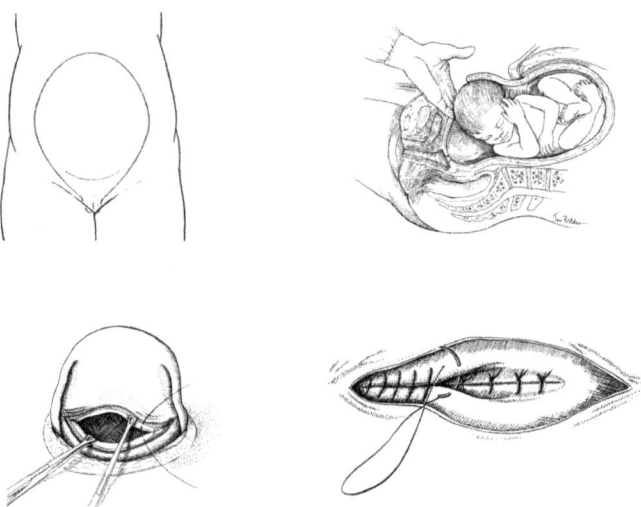

Post-operative Management

–Monitoring of vital signs and fundal status every 4-8 hours for 24 hours.

–Uterus massages and report extra lochia.

–Monitor fluids intake and output every four hours for 24 hours.

–Encourage early activity.

–Give fluids and soft diet after 6 hours.

–Antibiotics if indicated.

–Pain relief medication.

–If infant cord blood indicates Rh incompatibility, administer anti-Rh immunoglobulin.

–Discuss infant feeding and contraception.

REFERENCES

– Abalos E, Duley L, Steyn D. Antihypertensive drug therapy for mild to moderate hypertension during pregnancy. Cochrane Database Syst Rev 2014; 2: CD002252.

– Abdul-Kadir R, McLintock C, Ducloy A, et al. Evaluation and management of postpartum hemorrhage: consensus from an international expert panel. Transfusion 2014; 54: 1756.

– Alfirevic Z, Kelly A, Dowswell T. Intravenous oxytocin alone for cervical ripening and induction of labour. Cochrane Database Syst Rev 2009: CD003246.

– Alfirevic Z, Stampalija T, Gyte G. Fetal and umbilical Doppler ultrasound in high-risk pregnancies. Cochrane Database Syst Rev 2013; 11: CD007529.

– American College of Obstetricians and Gynecologists. Practice Bulletin no. 19: Thromboembolism in pregnancy. ACOG 2000; Washington, DC.

– American College of Obstetricians and Gynecologists. Practice Bulletin no. 76: Postpartum hemorrhage. Obstet Gynecol 2006; 108: 1039.

American College of Obstetricians and Gynecologists. Practice Bulletin no. 106: Intrapartum fetal heart rate monitoring: nomenclature, interpretation, and general management principles. Obstet Gynecol 2009; 114: 192.

– American College of Obstetricians and Gynecologists. Practice Bulletin no. 107: Induction of labor. Obstet Gynecol 2009; 114: 386.

– American College of Obstetricians and Gynecologists. Practice Bulletin no. 127: Management of preterm labor. Obstet Gynecol 2012; 119: 1308.

– American College of Obstetricians and Gynecologists. Practice Bulletin no. 134: Fetal growth restriction. Obstet Gynecol 2013; 121: 1122.

– Apantaku O, Mulik V. Maternal intra-partum fever. J Obstet Gynaecol 2007; 27: 12.

– Baacke K, Edwards R. Preinduction cervical assessment. Clin Obstet Gynecol 2006; 49: 564.

– Baschat A, Galan H, Bhide A, et al. Doppler and biophysical assessment in growth restricted fetuses: distribution of test results. Ultrasound Obstet Gynecol 2006; 27: 41.

– Baschat A. Fetal growth restriction - from observation to intervention. J Perinat Med 2010; 38: 239.

– Bashiri A, Burstein E, Bar-David J, et al. Face and brow presentation: independent risk factors. J Matern Fetal Neonatal Med 2008; 21: 357.

– Berghella V, Baxter J, Chauhan S. Evidence-based surgery for cesarean delivery. Am J Obstet Gynecol 2005; 193: 1607.

– Bricker L, Luckas M. Amniotomy alone for induction of labour. Cochrane Database Syst Rev 2000: CD002862.

– Chauhan S, Taylor M, Shields D, et al. Intrauterine growth restriction and oligohydramnios among high-risk patients. Am J Perinatol 2007; 24: 215.

– Cosmi E, Ambrosini G, D'Antona D, et al. Doppler, cardiotocography, and biophysical profile changes in growth-restricted fetuses. Obstet Gynecol 2005; 106: 1240.

– Dildy G. Postpartum hemorrhage: new management options. Clin Obstet Gynecol 2002; 45: 330.

– Figueras F, Gardosi J. Intrauterine growth restriction: new concepts in antenatal surveillance, diagnosis, and management. Am J Obstet Gynecol 2011; 204: 288.

– Gardberg M, Leonova Y, Laakkonen E. Malpresentations--impact on mode of delivery. Acta Obstet Gynecol Scand 2011; 90: 540.

– Gherman R, Chauhan S, Ouzounian J, et al. Shoulder dystocia: the unpreventable obstetric emergency with empiric management guidelines. Am J Obstet Gynecol 2006; 195: 657.

– Grivell R, Wong L, Bhatia V. Regimens of fetal surveillance for impaired fetal growth. Cochrane Database Syst Rev 2012; 6: CD007113.

– Gülmezoglu A, Crowther C, Middleton P, et al. Induction of labour for improving birth outcomes for women at or beyond term. Cochrane Database Syst Rev 2012; 6: CD004945.

– Gülmezoglu A, Hofmeyr G. Maternal nutrient supplementation for suspected impaired fetal growth. Cochrane Database Syst Rev 2000: CD000148.

– Gurewitsch E, Kim E, Yang J, et al. Comparing McRoberts' and Rubin's maneuvers for initial management of shoulder dystocia: an objective evaluation. Am J Obstet Gynecol 2005; 192: 153.

– Haas D, Imperiale T, Kirkpatrick P, et al. Tocolytic therapy: a meta-analysis and decision analysis. Obstet Gynecol 2009; 113: 585.

– Hecher K, Bilardo C, Stigter R, et al. Monitoring of fetuses with intrauterine growth restriction: a longitudinal study. Ultrasound Obstet Gynecol 2001; 18: 564.

– Hoffman M, Bailit J, Branch D, et al. A comparison of obstetric maneuvers for the acute management of shoulder dystocia. Obstet Gynecol 2011; 117: 1272.

– Howarth G, Botha D. Amniotomy plus intravenous oxytocin for induction of labour. Cochrane Database Syst Rev 2001: CD003250.

– Kramer M, Berg C, Abenhaim H, et al. Incidence, risk factors, and temporal trends in severe postpartum hemorrhage. Am J Obstet Gynecol 2013; 209: 449.

– Lausman A, McCarthy F, Walker M, et al. Screening, diagnosis, and management of intrauterine growth restriction. J Obstet Gynaecol Can 2012; 34: 17.

– Leduc D, Biringer A, Lee L, et al. Induction of labour. J Obstet Gynaecol Can 2013; 35: 840.

– Menticoglou S. A modified technique to deliver the posterior arm in severe shoulder dystocia. Obstet Gynecol 2006; 108: 755.

– Mozurkewich E, Chilimigras J, Koepke E, et al. Indications for induction of labour: a best-evidence review. BJOG 2009; 116: 626.

– Nakling J, Backe B. Pregnancy risk increases from 41 weeks of gestation. Acta Obstet Gynecol Scand 2006; 85: 663.

– Poggi S, Allen R, Patel C, et al. Randomized trial of McRoberts versus lithotomy positioning to decrease the force that is applied to the fetus during delivery. Am J Obstet Gynecol 2004; 191: 874.

– Poggi S, Spong C, Allen R. Prioritizing posterior arm delivery during severe shoulder dystocia. Obstet Gynecol 2003; 101: 1068.

– Resnik R. Intrauterine growth restriction. Obstet Gynecol 2002; 99: 490.

– Saccone G, Berghella V. Induction of labor at full term in uncomplicated singleton gestations: a systematic review and metaanalysis of randomized controlled trials. Am J Obstet Gynecol 2015; 213: 629.

– Sagi-Dain L, Sagi S. The role of episiotomy in prevention and management of shoulder dystocia: a systematic review. Obstet Gynecol Surv 2015; 70: 354.

– Smith J, Merrill D. Oxytocin for induction of labor. Clin Obstet Gynecol 2006; 49:594.

– Spain J, Frey H, Tuuli M, et al. Neonatal morbidity associated with shoulder dystocia maneuvers. Am J Obstet Gynecol 2015; 212: 353.

– Tapisiz O, Aytan H, Altinbas S, et al. Face presentation at term: a forgotten issue. J Obstet Gynaecol Res 2014; 40: 1573.

– Werner E, Savitz D, Janevic T, et al. Mode of delivery and neonatal outcomes in preterm, small-for-gestational-age newborns. Obstet Gynecol 2012; 120: 560.

– Westhoff G, Cotter A, Tolosa J. Prophylactic oxytocin for the third stage of labour to prevent postpartum haemorrhage. Cochrane Database Syst Rev 2013; 10: CD001808.

– Wetta L, Szychowski J, Seals S, et al. Risk factors for uterine atony/postpartum hemorrhage requiring treatment after vaginal delivery. Am J Obstet Gynecol 2013; 209: 51.

– Williams Obstetrics, 23rd Ed, Cunningham F, Leveno K, Bloom J, et al (Eds), McGraw-Hill, 2010.

www.ingramcontent.com/pod-product-compliance
Lightning Source LLC
Chambersburg PA
CBHW060411190526
45169CB00002B/859